UTERINE FIBROID SURGERY NUTRITION

Empowering Your Healing Journey And Understanding Surgical Solutions For Female Health

DR LUCAS KAYCE

DISCLAIMER

This book about illness and nutrition is not meant to replace expert medical advice, diagnosis, or treatment; rather, it is meant purely for informational reasons. This book's content is founded on broad concepts and recommendations for managing diseases and nutrition.

Before adopting any major dietary or lifestyle changes, readers are recommended to speak with a qualified healthcare provider, such as a licensed physician or registered dietitian, especially if they have pre-existing medical concerns. Everybody has different health demands, so what works for one person might not work for another.

The use of the information provided in this book may have unfavorable repercussions or consequences, for which the author and publisher disclaim all liability. No disease is meant to be identified, treated, cured, or prevented by the information provided.

The book may include contain references to medical literature or research findings; however readers are urged to independently confirm this material and contact reliable sources.

It is important to remember that the fields of nutrition and medicine are always changing, and that new findings could have an impact on the advice offered in this book. As a result, readers are urged to keep up with the most recent advancements in healthcare and, when in doubt, seek professional counsel.

By reading this book, readers agree that they are in charge of their own health decisions and release the author and publisher from any liability arising from the use of the material in the book, whether direct or indirect.

TABLE OF CONTENTS

ABOUT THE BOOK

The book "Uterine Fibroid Surgery Nutrition" is very important since it offers a thorough manual for those navigating the difficulties related to uterine fibroids and surgery. The information is carefully arranged to cover important topics, starting with a thorough introduction to uterine fibroids. In addition to providing readers with a thorough overview of these disorders, this part explores their etiology, risk factors, symptoms, and diagnostic techniques.

The book's main focus is on the many uterine fibroid surgery options, such as myomectomy, hysterectomy, and minimally invasive techniques. Every surgical strategy is broken down, giving clarity and understanding of the various possibilities. But what makes this book special is how much attention it pays to how important nutrition is for uterine fibroid surgery. The pre-surgery section provides comprehensive information on the significance of nutrition, including dietary advice and recommended supplements.

This information enables individuals to take an active role in their pre-surgery health.

The book shifts its focus to the crucial stage of recuperation, going beyond surgery. Nutritional tactics are described, including foods that promote healing, post-surgery dietary guidelines, and the importance of hydration in the healing process. The book also discusses using nutrition to control symptoms, including pain and discomfort and examines the role that nutrition plays in maintaining hormonal balance.

Understanding that maintaining long-term health requires a holistic approach, the book covers lifestyle modifications that are necessary for long-term well-being. The information gives readers a road map for navigating life after surgery and leading a healthier lifestyle, covering topics like stress management strategies, exercise's effect on uterine fibroids, and keeping a healthy weight.

A portion of the book devoted to dishes designed specifically for uterine fibroids enhances the usability of the book even more. Smoothies packed with nutrients, therapeutic salads and soups, and well-balanced meals for recuperation are offered, giving the dietary tactics covered in the book a practical and useful twist. All things considered, "Uterine Fibroid Surgery Nutrition" is an invaluable resource that provides a comprehensive approach that combines medical knowledge with useful dietary advice for those who are having or are thinking about having uterine fibroids removed.

AN OVERVIEW OF FIBROIDS IN WOMEN

Uterine fibroids are noncancerous growths that originate in the uterus and are also referred to as leiomyomas or myomas. These tumors can range in size from tiny, pea-sized nodules to bigger growths that can greatly expand the uterus. They are composed of muscle and fibrous tissue. Although the specific cause of uterine fibroids is unknown, certain lifestyle choices, genetic predispositions, and hormone fluctuations may all play a role in their growth. Women with uterine fibroids often have pelvic pain, heavy monthly flow, and pressure on the bladder or rectum, among other symptoms. This disorder is particularly common in fertile women. Medical, surgical, and lifestyle therapies are frequently used in conjunction with the diagnosis and treatment of uterine fibroids.

The role of surgery is one of the most important factors to take into account when treating uterine fibroids.

Surgical procedures might be advised to treat problems brought on by the growth of fibroids, relieve symptoms, or maintain fertility, among other reasons. Myomectomy, which removes the fibroids without destroying the uterus, and hysterectomy, which removes the uterus entirely, are common surgical treatments for uterine fibroids. The patient's reproductive goals, the size and location of the fibroids, the intensity of their symptoms, and other factors all play a role in the choice to have surgery.

NUTRITION IS CRUCIAL FOR UTERINE FIBROID SURGERY

The significance of nutrition in the context of uterine fibroid surgery cannot be emphasized. Sufficient diet is essential for accelerating recuperation, reducing difficulties after surgery, and readying the body for surgery. A diet that is well-balanced and abundant in vital nutrients, vitamins, and minerals is crucial for promoting overall well-being and aiding in the body's healing processes.

Before uterine fibroid surgery, nutritional concerns could include maintaining a healthy weight to lower the chance of surgical complications, maximizing iron levels to prevent anemia, and making sure you're getting enough vitamin C to repair wounds.

Furthermore, hormonal balance—which is intimately associated with the initiation and progression of uterine fibroids—can be impacted by nutrition. Some dietary decisions, such as eating a diet heavy in fruits and vegetables and low in red meat, may help maintain hormonal balance and maybe slow the growth of fibroids. Preoperative nutrition is also critically important for incorporating anti-inflammatory foods and staying hydrated, as these can help reduce inflammation and boost the body's immune response.

Uterine fibroids are a common and complicated health issue that affects women, requiring a multimodal approach to diagnosis and treatment. Surgical procedures like myomectomy and hysterectomy are frequently taken into consideration depending on the specifics of each case. But in the context of uterine fibroid surgery, the importance of nutrition should not be understated. A diet rich in nutrients and well-rounded not only helps the body cope with the demands of surgery but also improves general health and may even slow the progression of fibroid growth. A complete strategy for best results arises as medical personnel and patients work through the complexities of uterine fibroids. This holistic approach incorporates surgical competence and nutritional concerns.

CHAPTER ONE

KNOWING ABOUT UTERINE FIBROIDS

WHY DO UTERINE FIBROIDS OCCUR?

Known by other names, such as leiomyomas or myomas, uterine fibroids are noncancerous growths of the uterus that often develop during the childbearing years. Muscle cells and other tissues grow inside the uterine wall to form these tumors. Even while most uterine fibroids are benign, or not malignant, some women may nevertheless have a range of symptoms and consequences from them.

REASONS AND DANGER ELEMENTS

Although the precise etiology of uterine fibroids is yet unknown, several risk factors may be involved in their development. Hormones, namely progesterone and estrogen, are important in the development of fibroids. Given that women who have a family history of fibroids are more prone to get them, genetic factors appear to be involved as well.

Ethnicity also seems to have a role; Black women are more likely than women of other races to develop fibroids. Age is another risk factor; fibroids are more common in women in their 30s and 40s. Obesity is another risk factor; being overweight can accelerate the growth and development of fibroids.

SIGNS AND PROGNOSIS

Women with uterine fibroids might have a wide range of symptoms, and some may not even show any signs at all. Prolonged menstrual cycles, pelvic pain or pressure, excessive menstrual blood, trouble emptying the bladder, and constipation are common symptoms. Leg or back discomfort may also occasionally result from fibroids. A study of the patient's medical history, a pelvic exam, and imaging tests like MRIs and ultrasounds are often used to diagnose uterine fibroids. A medical professional might also suggest further testing, like a biopsy or hysteroscopy, to rule out other possible etiologies of the symptoms and confirm the existence of fibroids.

It is noteworthy that although uterine fibroids are prevalent, therapy is not always necessary for them. In cases where women exhibit minimal symptoms or none at all, a cautious waiting strategy could be advised. However, there are several therapy alternatives available for those who have severe symptoms or problems.

These could include hormone therapy to reduce the size of the fibroids, painkillers to control menstrual flow, or surgical procedures like hysterectomy or myomectomy to remove the uterus or fibroids.

To sum up, to comprehend uterine fibroids, one must acknowledge that they are uterine growths that are not cancerous and can impact fertile women. Their growth is influenced by several factors, including age, ethnicity, hormones, and genetics, however, the precise causes are yet unknown.

A mix of medical history, pelvic exams, and imaging tests are used in the diagnosing process, which can encompass mild to severe symptoms.

Depending on the severity of the symptoms, several treatment options are available, such as medication, hormone therapy, surgery, or careful waiting. To choose the best course of action for their unique situation, women must collaborate closely with their healthcare providers.

CHAPTER TWO

DIFFERENT UTERINE FIBROID SURGERY TYPES

MYOMECTOMY

A myomectomy is a surgical operation used to remove fibroids from the uterus while leaving it intact. Women who want to avoid having a full hysterectomy or preserve their fertility frequently consider this strategy. A myomectomy can be carried out using a variety of methods, such as a laparoscopic, hysteroscopic, or abdominal procedure. Larger or more numerous fibroids can be removed using an abdominal myomectomy, which requires making an incision in the abdominal wall to reach the fibroids. Small incisions are made during a minimally invasive laparoscopic myomectomy operation, and a camera-guided device is used to remove the fibroids. When it comes to submucosal fibroids that extend into the uterine cavity, hysteroscopic myomectomy is the best option for removing the tumors through the cervix.

HYSTERECTOMY

A more drastic procedure called a hysterectomy involves completely removing the uterus and, in certain situations, the cervix. Since there is no chance of a fibroid recurrence after this treatment, it is regarded as a permanent cure for uterine fibroids. There are many hysterectomy operations, such as subtotal or partial hysterectomy, which removes only the uterus while leaving the cervix in place, and total hysterectomy, which removes both the uterus and the cervix. When other therapies have failed, hysterectomy may be advised in cases of significant fibroids or if symptoms are chronic. Although it is a useful option, its effects on fertility and general health must be taken into account, therefore it is typically saved for situations in which maintaining fertility is not a top priority.

LITTLE-INVASIVE TECHNIQUES

Because they provide patients with faster recovery times and fewer difficulties than traditional open surgeries, minimally invasive treatments are becoming more and more popular for treating uterine fibroids. Small incisions are made during these procedures, such as laparoscopic and robotic-assisted operations, and specialized equipment is utilized to remove or destroy the fibroids. Another minimally invasive procedure is uterine artery embolizations (UAE), which involves injecting microscopic particles into the blood vessels supplying the fibroids to cause them to contract. Focused ultrasound waves are used in Magnetic Resonance-guided Focused Ultrasound Surgery, a non-invasive method, to heat and kill fibroids. Women who would prefer a shorter recovery period or who wish to avoid a major surgery may consider these minimally invasive procedures.

A patient's overall health, desired fertility, and the size and location of their fibroids all play a role in the decision to have uterine fibroid surgery. When more drastic action is needed, hysterectomy is taken into consideration, although myomectomy is preferred for people who want to preserve their fertility.

Alternatives that strike a compromise between effectiveness, less invasiveness, and quicker recovery are provided by minimally intrusive techniques. In the end, a detailed discussion between the patient and her healthcare provider—which takes into consideration unique circumstances and treatment goals—should be the basis for choosing a particular surgical procedure.

CHAPTER THREE

GETTING READY FOR SURGERY ON UTERINE FIBROIDS

THE VALUE OF EATING WELL BEFORE SURGERY

It's imperative to prepare for uterine fibroid surgery in a way that will maximize results and support general health while recovering. Understanding how important nutrition is before surgery is a crucial part of this preparation. A nutritious, well-balanced diet is essential for promoting wound healing, boosting immunity, and lowering the chance of problems.

Before having surgery for uterine fibroids, people should concentrate on eating a diet high in vital nutrients. Since proteins are the building blocks of cells and are essential to the healing process, consuming an adequate amount of protein is essential for tissue repair and recovery. Including lean protein sources like fish, poultry, tofu, and beans can help the body heal from the previous surgery.

A diet rich in fruits and vegetables not only offers protein but also important vitamins, minerals, and antioxidants. These nutrients play a critical role in improving general health, decreasing inflammation, and strengthening the immune system. Antioxidants in particular improve the body's ability to withstand the stress of surgery by shielding cells from damage caused by free radicals.

DIETARY GUIDELINES

Before undergoing uterine fibroid surgery, dietary guidelines stress the significance of staying well-hydrated. Many biological processes, such as blood volume maintenance, temperature regulation, and renal support, depend on adequate hydration. Maintaining enough hydration levels can also help avoid frequent post-surgery issues like constipation and urinary tract infections.

Reducing the consumption of specific foods, such as processed sweets and foods heavy in sodium, can help lower the risk of problems following surgery.

Diets high in sodium can cause blood pressure and fluid retention, and diets high in sugar can harm the immune system and metabolic health in general. An easier recovery process can be achieved in the weeks preceding surgery by eating a balanced, low-inflammatory diet.

SUPPLEMENTS FOR NUTRITION

Supplemental nutrition may also help the body get ready for surgery to remove uterine fibroids. It is essential to speak with medical professionals to ascertain particular requirements and prevent prescription interactions. Iron, zinc, and vitamin C are common supplements advised before surgery since they are vital for wound healing and immune system maintenance.

Understanding the significance of nutrition is a key component of a comprehensive strategy for uterine fibroid surgical preparation. A well-balanced, nutrient-rich diet, along with the consideration of appropriate nutritional supplements, will help ensure the best possible preoperative health. Setting these priorities first aids in laying the groundwork for a successful surgical procedure and promotes a quicker healing period.

CHAPTER FOUR

DIETARY TECHNIQUES FOR HEALING

POST-SURGERY DIETARY GUIDELINES

Following surgery, a healthy diet is essential to the healing process. Adhering to particular dietary guidelines is crucial for promoting recovery and general health. People may have changes in their appetite, digestion, and absorption of nutrients in the first post-surgery phase. A diet that is well-balanced and customized for each person is necessary to address these issues.

Post-surgery, it is especially crucial to emphasize a high-protein diet because protein is essential for tissue repair and cell regeneration. Fish, poultry, eggs, and beans are examples of lean protein foods that can aid in tissue repair and hasten healing.

Incorporating enough healthy fats and carbohydrates also gives the body the energy it needs to repair and rebuild strength.

Prioritizing micronutrients like vitamins and minerals is also advised because they are crucial for wound healing and immune system function. During the healing stage, vitamins A, C, and E as well as minerals zinc and selenium are especially helpful. A post-surgical dietary plan can be specifically tailored to satisfy nutritional demands based on the type of operation and the patient's health status by consulting with a healthcare expert or a registered dietitian.

FOODS TO ENCOURAGE HEALING

A few foods have a reputation for promoting healing and can help with the healing process following surgery. Including a range of foods high in nutrients can give the body the building blocks it needs to heal and regenerate damaged tissue. Vitamins A and C are abundant in dark leafy greens, like spinach and kale, and they support the production of collagen and the immune system.

Antioxidants found in fruits like berries and citrus fruits help fight oxidative stress and inflammation, creating an environment that is favorable for healing.

The anti-inflammatory qualities of omega-3 fatty acids, which are present in fatty fish like salmon and mackerel, may help to lessen post-surgery inflammation and speed up the healing process.

Consuming foods high in fiber, vitamins, and minerals—such as whole grains, nuts, and seeds—supports digestive health and general healing. Dairy products and their fortified plant-based substitutes can also be excellent providers of calcium and vitamin D, which are essential for healthy bones, particularly following orthopedic procedures.

HYDRATION AND ITS FUNCTION IN RECOVERY

Keeping enough fluids in the body is essential to the healing process following surgery. Water is necessary for several physiological processes, including waste removal, temperature regulation, and the movement of nutrients. Dehydration can impair blood flow and nutrient delivery to the surgery site, which might hinder the body's capacity to heal.

Sufficient water also helps avoid issues like constipation, which are frequently experienced after surgery as a result of altered eating and activity habits. People should try to drink the recommended amount of fluids, which can include clear broths, herbal teas, and water. It's crucial to heed any specific advice given by medical specialists, though, as some medical conditions or surgical procedures may call for different fluid intake regimens.

It's important to keep an eye on one's level of hydration, and people should be aware of symptoms like dry mouth or dark urine. Although it's critical to maintain hydration, consuming too many fluids can also cause electrolyte imbalances. Maintaining equilibrium and making sure you're always at a somewhat high level of hydration are key components of a successful recovery process.

CHAPTER FIVE

CONTROLLING SYMPTOMS WITH FOOD

RELIEVING PAIN AND SORENESS:

An essential component of diet-based symptom management is effectively treating pain and discomfort. For people with a variety of medical illnesses, specific dietary decisions can be quite important in reducing these symptoms. Anti-inflammatory foods have been demonstrated to lower inflammation and help with pain reduction. Examples of these foods include berries, leafy green vegetables, and fatty fish high in omega-3 fatty acids. Furthermore, adding natural anti-inflammatory spices to food, such as ginger and turmeric, can offer a comprehensive approach to pain management.

Moreover, keeping a diet that is well-balanced and includes enough vitamins and minerals is crucial for good health and may help with symptom relief. For example, foods high in magnesium, such as whole grains, nuts, and seeds, have been linked to pain relief and muscle relaxation. In addition to supporting joint health and assisting with the appropriate operation of body systems, hydration is essential for the effective management of discomfort. Drinking enough water throughout the day can be a straightforward yet powerful tactic for people looking to reduce their pain and discomfort.

HORMONE BALANCING THROUGH DIET

The regulation of hormonal balance in the body is significantly influenced by nutrition. A variety of symptoms, such as mood swings, exhaustion, and irregular menstrual cycles, can be attributed to hormonal imbalances. A diet rich in nutrients and low in processed foods that can upset the endocrine system is the way to choose for hormonal wellness. A diet rich in fruits, vegetables, and whole grains can supply vital vitamins and minerals to support the production and balance of hormones.

Broccoli, kale, and Brussels sprouts are examples of cruciferous vegetables. These vegetables include chemicals that support estrogen metabolism and help maintain hormonal balance. Hormone production can also be supported by consuming healthy fats like those in nuts, avocados, and olive oil. Flaxseeds and fatty fish are good sources of omega-3 fatty acids, which have been associated with better hormone regulation and may help those with hormonal abnormalities.

Sustaining steady blood sugar levels is another essential component of hormonal equilibrium. Foods high in fiber, complex carbs, and protein can help stabilize blood sugar levels and reduce swings that could affect hormone levels. All things considered, a balanced and nutrient-dense diet is an essential tactic for those trying to properly balance their hormones and treat related ailments.

CHAPTER SIX

MODIFICATIONS TO LIFESTYLE FOR LONG-TERM HEALTH

SUSTAINING A HEALTHY WEIGHT

Long-term health is fundamentally dependent on maintaining a healthy weight. It has significant effects on general well-being and goes beyond aesthetic issues. A balanced diet, consistent exercise, and mindful eating are the keys to reaching and maintaining a healthy weight. Maintaining the proper balance aids in preventing several illnesses, including diabetes, cardiovascular disease, and joint disorders. It's critical to adopt a realistic and sustainable strategy to weight control, avoiding fad diets and quick solutions in favor of small, long-term improvements."

THE EFFECTS OF EXERCISE ON UTERINE FIBROIDS

Long-term health promotion is greatly aided by exercise, which has benefits that go beyond physical fitness. Exercise has been connected to the management of uterine fibroids when it comes to women's health specifically. Frequent exercise can aid in blood circulation improvement, inflammation reduction, and hormone regulation—all of which are variables that contribute to the onset and growth of uterine fibroids. Combining aerobic, strength, and flexibility training into one's routine not only helps one lose weight but also has a good impact on hormone balance, which may reduce the incidence of uterine fibroids.

TECHNIQUES FOR STRESS MANAGEMENT

Since chronic stress can have a significant negative impact on one's physical and mental health, stress management strategies are essential to preserving one's long-term health. Numerous medical disorders, such as digestive problems, immune system damage, and cardiovascular diseases, have been linked to stress. Chronic stress may also make diseases like uterine fibroids worse for women's health. Using practical stress-reduction techniques, including yoga, deep breathing exercises, mindfulness meditation, or taking up a hobby, can help reduce stress and encourage balance. In addition to improving mental health, these behaviors are essential in delaying the onset or aggravation of stress-related illnesses.

Modifying one's lifestyle for the long term requires a comprehensive strategy that includes keeping a healthy weight, exercising frequently, and using productive stress-reduction methods. These components work together to promote general well-being because they are interrelated. Adopting a balanced lifestyle can help people avoid many health problems and improve their quality of life over time. It's critical to understand that these adjustments are long-term, sustainable, and the first steps toward living a happier, healthier life.

CHAPTER SEVEN

RECIPES FOR THE HEALTH OF UTERINE FIBROIDS

RICH IN NUTRIENTS SMOOTHIES

Smoothies that are high in nutrients can be a tasty and healthy method to boost your general well-being when it comes to uterine fibroid health. You may make these smoothies using a wide variety of fruits, vegetables, and other high-nutrient items. Antioxidant-rich berries like strawberries and blueberries are well known for their ability to reduce inflammation and oxidative stress brought on by uterine fibroids. Leafy greens like kale and spinach offer a lot of vitamins, minerals, and fiber to your smoothies, which helps maintain digestive health.

Smoothies can be made more nutritious by adding nuts and seeds, such as almonds, chia seeds, and flaxseeds, in addition to fruits and vegetables. These seeds help maintain hormonal balance and provide anti-inflammatory properties since they are high in fiber and omega-3 fatty acids. Smoothies with added protein can benefit from the addition of yogurt, nut butter, or plant-based protein powder. This promotes general vitality and muscular recuperation in addition to offering a fulfilling and energizing beverage.

Soups and salads that are healing: Rich in nutrients and simple to digest, soups and salads that are healing are essential to maintaining the health of uterine fibroids. Including a range of vibrant veggies in salads guarantees a varied selection of antioxidants, vitamins, and minerals. Because leafy greens like kale and arugula have a high fiber content that facilitates digestion and increases feelings of fullness, they can be very healthy.

Selecting broth-based soups that feature a variety of veggies and lean proteins can be calming and nourishing when it comes to healing soups. The addition of turmeric, ginger, and garlic to soups enhances their taste and imparts anti-inflammatory qualities that may help alleviate uterine fibroid symptoms. Furthermore, using whole grains in salads, such as brown rice or quinoa, offers a nutritious supply of carbs that promote long-lasting energy and general well-being.

PROPER MEALS FOR RECUPERATION

Maintaining a healthy, well-balanced diet is essential for recovering from uterine fibroids. Lean meats, complete grains, healthy fats, and an assortment of fruits and vegetables should all be included in a balanced diet. Lean proteins, including those found in fish, poultry, tofu, and lentils, support general recovery by aiding in muscle maintenance and tissue regeneration.

Whole grains with high fiber content, such as brown rice, quinoa, and oats, enhance digestive health and offer a consistent release of energy. Including healthy fats from foods like nuts, avocados, and olive oil helps maintain hormonal balance and satiety. A varied intake of vital vitamins and minerals is ensured by including a vibrant assortment of fruits and vegetables.

Furthermore, since water is essential for both detoxification and general body processes, maintaining proper hydration is critical to recovery. Reducing the amount of processed food, refined sugar, and caffeine can also help to create a more well-rounded and supportive diet for the health of uterine fibroids. To put it briefly, for those who are managing uterine fibroids, embracing a holistic approach to nutrition with an emphasis on nutrient-rich foods can be quite important in supporting healing and overall well-being.